10 Bags
a Sunflower Hat

Leslee Wlodyka

10 Bags and a Sunflower Hat

All scripture quotations in this book, except those noted otherwise, are from the Holy Bible, New International Version. Copyright © 1973, 1978, 1984 by International Bible Society. Used by permission of Zondervan Publishing House.

Library of Congress Number: 2008942620
ISBN: 978-1-60126-160-1

Masthof Press
*219 Mill Road
Morgantown, PA 19543-9516
www.masthof.com*

Dedication

To my daughter, Brynn, who was my balance
and to my daughter, Bree, who is my soul responsibility.

Contents

Author's Note

I am writing this book because I like to be prepared. I am very organized and I have the sorry/unfortunate ability to remember trivia. Among some pieces of trivia, I occasionally find diamonds in the rough, knowledge that, when I make sense of it, can help my family, friends and patients. This book is being created for that purpose, to help put together all the pieces of knowledge, or trivia, as I like to call it, that I have collected. I am hoping that when I, myself, have dementia this book will make it possible for my family to know what to expect and what to do, when I am no longer the person they remember. There is always a change in life circumstances and it should be handled in a certain manner to increase coping.

For me, the change will be waiting for someone to give me my big, straw sunflower gardening hat and ten purses, as I would need five for each arm. Then I would hope that they would let me wander about collecting the flowers that no one but I can see. The organized trivia in this book should be used to help family and friends of patients with dementia to understand why this happens, in simple terms, and to provide them with strategies for coping.

Leslee Wlodyka

Acknowledgements

Where do I begin to thank all who have helped me?

To the nursing staff at The Reading Hospital and Medical Center, Spruce Pavilion, who, when I said let's try sensory integration techniques, looked at me as if I had lost my mind and needed to be there as a patient, instead they tried anyway.

To the psychiatrists of Spruce Pavillian who helped me create a sensory room with donations from their own pockets, thank you.

To Martha Connelly LCSW, director of the Willows Program, thanks does not seem like enough. You pushed me into speaking. You gave me the confidence to continue when I thought it just wasn't going the way I thought it should go and backed me more than once, I am sure, with the administration. You are a brave woman.

To Mary Jo Brown MA, NCL, LPC, the director of the Paws for Wellness Program at The Reading Hospital and my boss, for her diplomacy. I know I am abrasive. She has on more than one occasion gone to bat with my co-workers again, thank you for your support.

To Christine Leinbach, for being my partner in crime and for some reason never getting the same billing for the work we do together in the Willows Program, thanks.

And last but not least to Savannah and Joan for their patience. They both took my thoughts that are organized in my head but become jumbled when coming from my mouth and made them orgainized again. Thank you to Savannah for her writing experience and Joan for her Pediatric Occupational Therapy experience.

Introduction

There is a poem by Bernice McCarthy from her book, *About Learning* (2000), which details the sensory integration of a child. The poem found in *About Learning* parallels changes within the demented geriatric population, but in an opposite direction.

> Watch any child learn,
> even the youngest,
> perhaps especially the youngest.
> What does this child do?
> Enters into & absorbs by what is.
> Looks within.
> Looks without.
> Feels,
> puzzles,
> tries,
> owns -
> learns.
> Not yet contaminated by fear of failures,
> not yet anxious about grades.
> When you watch a child learn,
> The dynamic is apparent.

Two major things happen –
The child experiences,
And the child reacts to experience.
Reality greets the child
And the child greets reality.
The child is and the child does.
So the pattern of being someone,
Then reacting to the world as that someone,
Happens over and over.
This is the learning cycle (5).

The opposite way of reacting can be seen in the elderly. The elderly are afraid to interact and have difficulty absorbing and interpreting information. Their eyes have difficulty looking within, for their vision fails them. Feelings have become numb in geriatric dementia patients. Parts of the brain no longer puzzle, or even try to interpret anything, in many geriatric dementia patients. Also, most of their ownership is gone, however, they can still learn with a great deal of repetition. McCarthy (2000) wrote, "So the pattern of being someone, then reacting to the world as that someone happens over and over" (5).

I hope that this book speaks for itself, but if it does not manage to do so, the things that are needed to go through the stages of dementia would be fit into these ten bags:

Bag One—Exercise: With exercise, balance is increased, the fear of falling is decreased and memory production is increased in the brain.

Bag Two—Socialization: Socialization inhibits isolation and allows a person to spend time with family and friends, enjoying what life has to offer.

Bag Three—Completion of simple tasks, such as setting the table: Completion of simple tasks allows a person to feel independent for as long as possible. Simplification of methods to care for basic needs allows a person to continue completion of ADLs so they can feel independent.

Bag Four—Relaxation: Relaxation promotes a higher ability to cope with a stressful situation.

Bag Five—Simplifying enjoyable tasks: Gardening and coloring, using markers or crayons to increase proprioception. Pens and pencils do not require the same pressure and remember many of us have a preference for either light pressure or weight.

Bag Six—Continuing to simplify basic self-care needs such as toileting and dressing: Simplification of basic needs allows a person to continue completion of ADLs so that they can feel independent.

Bag Seven—Sensory snacks, such as aromatherapy: "Sensory snacks" is a literal synonym for stopping to smell the roses, stopping to smell the coffee, stopping to feel the warmth of a day, or stopping to drink a cup of tea. In other words, enjoy the sensory pleasures that our environment allows for us.

Bag Eight—Make sure that their affairs are in order and all legal matters are taken care of, including choosing a durable power of attorney: Putting affairs in order and choosing a durable power of attorney makes it possible to have the help that is needed at the time it is required and takes extra stress off of the person. **Don't be in denial.**

Bag Nine—Remember the past: Reminisce. Remembrance shapes the present and the future.

Bag Ten—Respect: Respect all that you were, all that you are now and all that you will be.

CHAPTER 1

Exercise

While people understand that exercise will help to increase general health, build muscle strength and endurance, exercise also benefits the brain. In order to maintain a healthy brain, and more specifically a healthy hippocampus, exercise is an important part of a daily routine. When I initially started my 5-day-a-week, 45-minute, seated fitness program, it wasn't 45 minutes, but 20 minutes. I was afraid the elderly I worked with were too frail. Boy was I wrong! The people too frail were my young students! The program has evolved as I have evolved; just like life, it keeps changing.

Exercising both sides of the body equally charges up the endorphins, seratonin, and dopamine in the brain and sends it to the parts of the brain in need of motivation. The hippocampus improves memory because it helps the brain to recognize its environment. Moreover, exercise is also a great way to combat depression. The chemicals that help the hippocampus function better also help to eliminate depression and stimulate good feelings.

Patients with dementia revert back to their two natural fears: the fear of falling and the fear of noises.

Noise is relative. Loud noise during the day will scare anyone, but it is the small noises at night that set the typical mind to worrying. This kicks in the "fight or flight" response, and, for the demented person or the very depressed person, the increased stress can be disastrous.

The fear of falling can be helped by the vestibular system being more balanced. The external portion of the vestibular system can be found behind the right and left eardrums and the structures look like the planet Saturn in miniature form. They are made up of free-flowing crystals in a liquid. When a patient with dementia ceases to move around and exercise, the vestibular system can become unbalanced. The liquid begins to gel and does not allow the crystals their free flow, which causes the patient's balance to be compromised. The patients may begin to feel dizzy and nauseous. This will bring back their fear of falling. When a patient with dementia becomes unbalanced and dizzy they feel like they might fall. In order to help them regain their balance and calm their fear, they must begin movement. The best way for a geriatric dementia patient to regain their balance is through the activity of rocking. Rocking chairs and large porch swings create motion for the patient and this helps to return the vestibular system to its normal balanced state, thus relieving the dizziness and nausea.

Rocking in a safety rocking chair, or in a large porch swing, daily, greatly helps a geriatric dementia patient. By promoting balance to the body by keeping the liquid and crystals in the vestibular system free flowing through movement, the patient feels much more grounded. A balanced patient will feel the fear of falling much less than an unbalanced patient; therefore, it is recommended that geriatric dementia patients have movement in their daily lives.

Beyond basic movement like rocking, it has been discovered that other exercises are beneficial to people with dementia. Voltz (2005) stated, "Exercise can have an impact on several risk factors related to fall prevention, including gaining muscle strength and flexibility, increasing endurance, increasing bone density and improving self-confidence which can dissolve the fear of falling," (45). As exercise can help to calm the fear of falling, it can also help to keep the mind sharper. In addition to the chemicals, which are released into the brain during exercise, exercising in a group environment, according to Voltz (2005) "[enables] socialization and facilitation of self-confidence and self-awareness of ability," (45). Increased socialization leads to greater use of interpersonal skills.

At the University of Arizona, undergraduate students began a program to study the effects that exercise has on patients with dementia. They included in their study twenty-four patients with mild to moderate dementia. Through the course of the study the students worked one-on-one with the patients. As the patients were exercising, they were asked to do word associations, as well as to answer questions. The physical fitness portion of the study included stretching, treadmills and stationary bicycles, balance exercises, and two sets of ten to twelve repetitions on weight resistance machines. Arkin (2007) wrote of the exercise program, "Everyone was started at five minutes on the treadmill and five minutes on the bike with incremental increases as tolerated. . . . On the weight machines, repetitions were first increased from ten to twelve at a given weight. . . . Typically two pounds at a time for the upper body machines and ten to twenty pounds on the leg press" (62). As the patients exercised the students would talk to them. They would be asked to tell the students what they knew about John F. Kennedy, or to tell the students what they knew about Alzheimer's. According to Sharon Arkin's article in the *American Journal of Alzheimer's Disease & Other Dementia* (2007):

> "The language and memory stimulation activities administered provided practice in all of the important cognitive operations that have been identified as relevant to conversational performance and that are typically compromised in persons with [dementia]: attention, explicit memory, judgment and reasoning, planning, problem solving, set shifting, abstract reasoning, and semantic memory. Activities requiring deep concentration or attention to visual stimuli were administered during rest periods before after and between physical activities" (65).

This study yielded results, which pointed to a strong correlation between improved cognitive operations and language-enriched exercise programs. Also, according to Arkin (2007), "All four of the four-year completers were at the same . . . stage of dementia at the end of treatment as they were four years previously" (68). This means that the patients who took part in the four years of the study were able to stave off the long-term effects of dementia. Essentially, the patients were able to maintain the same level of cognitive operations that they had prior to taking part in the study, all of the way through the four years of the study. Moreover, it is important to note that Teri, McCurry, Bucher, Logsdon, LaCroix, Kukall, Barlow and Larson (1998) wrote that, "exercise into standard care practices for individuals with dementia appears relevant and feasible" (9).

It is important to keep exercise environments for patients with dementia multi-sensory. The use of natural light, comfortable temperature, and perhaps the soothing aroma of lavender, helps to keep the environment relaxed. Also, while it is important to keep the environment comfortable, it is also important to keep it free of distractions, so the use of a few plants might give the patients something to look at, without giving them too much distraction. Moreover, the use of distracting sounds should be avoided. The simple sound of the caregiver's voice is sufficient to complete the multisensory environment.

The activities used, should also be multisensory. Patricia Heyn (2003) reported, "Multisensory stimulation activities are defined as approaches and strategies that stimulate the primary senses in a focused manner to promote more adaptive behaviors or adaptive environments and generate enjoyable sensorial experiences. The sensory input is the stimuli reaching a person through sensory channels including arousal, olfactory, auditory, and touch" (248). The use of imagery and the use of storytelling are important to the multisensory approach. Heyn (2003) also wrote, "Storytelling is the process of narrating incidents, events and themes to stimulate engagement and participation in the rehabilitation, health and prevention process. . . . Imagery is the process of developing a mental representation of persons, objects, or feelings. Imagery evokes the stimulation and use of various senses" (248). Therefore, it is very important to make sure that a multisensory environment and multisensory stimulation are used in the exercise, socialization and communication of patients with dementia.

The blood flow to the brain, coupled with the proper flow of oxygen, help to keep the brain functioning properly. Exercise increases the blood flow to the brain and also increases oxygen intake. Once the blood flow and oxygen intake increase, so does appetite, which helps to keep the body healthy. It is also important to remember to remain relaxed and calm. At the end of exercising, patients should sit and relax, breathing deeply with their eyes closed, concentrating on breathing. It is also helpful if they massage their tempero-mandibular joint while they are breathing, with their eyes closed. This releases the tension from the jaw, which in turn releases the tension from the head and neck. Once the muscles in the neck are loosened, blood flows more quickly through the carotid arteries into the brain, and from the brain through the jugular vein. When a calm and relaxed state is obtained, the blood flows more freely and quickly to and from the brain, allowing the brain better functioning.

CHAPTER 2

Exercise and the Brain

*Please check with your physician
before beginning any exercise program.*

Leslee Wlodyka's exercise program can encompass everyone at every level. It allows for socialization of the patients as well. Her program can be done with two people, a caregiver and a demented patient, or with as many as fourteen people. She starts with a deep breathing exercise, breathing in through the nose and out through the mouth. This is done three or four times to increase oxygen levels. The reason for her exercise program is because it challenges both sides of the brain simultaneously, which charges up the hippocampus, which is the central part of the brain, and it controls memories and making sense of the environment. Exercise also produces three chemicals—seratonin, dopamine and endorphins. Endorphins make a person feel good and they also have a morphine-like effect. When Leslee exercises she trains in three areas. The first portion of exercise is to warm up. The second portion of exercise is a strengthening portion in which Leslee uses free weights, but is careful to not exceed three pounds of weight with her patients. The third portion of exercise is a cool down phase, in which she teaches relaxation and coping skills.

Leslee begins with the fingers and she tells her patients to play an imaginary piano for a minute to warm up the joints in the hands and the thumbs. The thumb exercises consist of circles, touching the thumb to the base of the little finger and then make a circle touching the thumb to all the fingers in order, starting with the index finger and progressing to the little finger. Do this ten repetitions. This creates a synovial fluid to cushion the joints. The following exercise is to touch the toes or the knees, depending on the patients' physical limitations. On Monday she begins with one touch to the toes or the knees and by Friday she has reached five touches to the toes or the knees. The next exercise is to make circles with the wrists moving both clockwise and counter-clockwise. As with the last exercise, Monday she begins with one set of wrist circles in each direction and by Friday she has reached three sets of wrist circles in each direction.

Following this exercise Leslee asks her patients to reach both arms out in front of them and to clasp their hands together, and keeping their hands clasped together, to move their hands toward their body and away from their body, so that their arms form what looks like a hoop. They do ten repetitions and then they switch the position. Their next position is similar to the first. Without unclasping the hands they turn their arms, so that the palms are facing away from the body and they repeat the first activity, by moving their hands toward and away from the body in ten repetitions. Next, they lift their clasped hands above their head and they move their hands towards and away from the top of their head in a set of ten repetitions. And finally, they do an exercise that Leslee calls, "chopping wood." They take their clasped hands and pretend that they are holding an ax and they bring their imaginary ax behind their head and then they bring it over their head and down in front of them, as though they were bringing the ax down on a piece of firewood. They do a set of ten repetitions of this exercise as well. All of these movements exercise the muscles in the arms, hands, shoulders and the back and increase synovial fluids. Also, keeping the arms strong is essential because the arms do all of our purposeful activity, such as eating, dressing ourselves, and grooming ourselves.

Leslee's next exercise is called, "paddling the canoe." In this exercise she has her patients clasp their hands together, pretending that they are holding a canoe paddle. They take their imaginary paddle and they do a deep stroke to one side of their body and then they do a deep stroke to the other side of their body. She asks each patient to do ten repetitions of this exercise. Next, they do the "hula dance," in which they move their hands from side to side as a hula dancer might. She does ten repetitions of this exercise. Finally, she asks her patients to sway like trees, which is an exercise in which she asks her patients to lift their arms in the air and to move them back and forth in a set of ten repetitions. These motions exercise the oblique muscles, the shoulders, the back and the arms.

Next, Leslee asks her patients to do shoulder shrugs, which loosen the shoulder and neck muscles and help to create blood flow to the brain. When a patient is tense or anxious, the first thing that they do is clench their teeth together. Next they begin to tighten the muscles in their neck and shoulders. The tightening of these muscles restricts the blood flow through the carotid artery and the jugular vein, which restricts the blood flow to the brain. In order to help relax the muscles in the shoulders and the next, Leslee has her patients do the shoulder shrugs. By allowing more blood to the brain, more activity in all parts of the brain can be sustained.

In order to exercise the vestibular system, Leslee asks her patients to "row the boat." Before the patients begin to row the boat, Leslee asks them to name a body of water, to stimulate their memory. In rowing the boat, each patient holds onto a covered theraband, as though it were a boat oar, and they rock back and forth with the theraband, as if they were rowing a boat. The rocking of the patients exercises their vestibular system, which helps with balance and decreases the fear of falling.

Next Leslee moves to the legs. She asks her patients to move their feet up and down at the ankles in a set of ten repetitions. Then she asks her patients to turn their toes in toward each other (unless they've had a hip injury or a hip surgery) and do the same exercise in a set of ten repetitions. Next, she has her patients turn their toes away from each other and do the same exercise in a set of ten repetitions. Finally, she asks her patients to make ankle circles in one direction ten times and then switching direction, to make another ten ankle circles. This exercise helps to keep blood flowing through the lower portion of the legs, where most blood clots occur.

To help stimulate the memory, Leslee asks her patients to name a mountain. Once a mountain has been named she asks her patients to march up the mountains. In this exercise they remain seated, but move their legs and march while seated, pounding their legs into the ground. Pounding the legs into the ground creates microscopic fractures in the bone, which creates bone density. When there is a done fracture, because of the build up of bone density, that particular piece of the bone will never fracture or break again. This helps fight osteoporosis.

The next exercise stretches the hamstring, which improves vision. If a patient can straighten their knees and walk looking forward, they are less likely to fall. However, bent knees have the patient looking down, making them more top-heavy and more likely to fall. If a person has had surgery on their hip or has had a hip injury, they should kick their legs out in front of them from their knees only. However, if a person does not have any hip injuries of any type or hip surgery they should kick their legs in front of them from their hip. This increases the strength of the lower abdominal muscles, which makes less work for the lower back muscles, which in turn, helps to decrease back problems.

Next, Leslee asks her patients to do whole leg circles to the left and whole leg circles to the right while seated. She does ten sets in each direction. This exercise improves the lower back abdominal muscles and the lower back muscles. This concludes the first part of Leslee's exercise program.

The second portion of Leslee's program is a strengthening portion with the use of free weights. The use of free weights increases proprioception, or the ability to identify where one body part is in relation to another body part. She uses small dumbbells, in one pound, two pounds, or three pounds. She never exceeds three pounds of free weight with her patients. In her first exercise she asks her standing patients to hold the weights at their side, keeping their shoulders relaxed and their muscles loosened. The patients, holding the free weights, then use their wrists only to move the dumbbells, first with their palms facing back, then with their palms facing toward their body, and finally with their palms facing upwards. They do repetitions of ten of each exercise on Monday. By Friday, Leslee asks her patients to increase the sets of ten repetitions from one set, to three sets if they are able.

Next Leslee asks her patients to do bicep curls. In the bicep curl, the patients' hands hang at their sides, their shoulders are loose and they bring their weights from their sides, to their shoulders and then back to their sides again. The patients do ten repetitions of this exercise. After the bicep curls, the patients do what Leslee calls, "the boxer." She asks her patients to name a famous boxer before they begin this exercise. In the boxer, each patient takes their weights in their hands and holds their hands at chest level. Then they push one hand outward away from their body and as they are bringing that hand back toward their body, they push their other hand away from their body. In this manner, they look like they are boxing. Through all of this Leslee asks her patients to count with her so that she knows that they are breathing. She asks that they do ten repetitions of "the boxer."

Next, she asks her patients to hold their arms outstretched on each side of their body, with their weights in their hands, palms down. The patients then move their arms up and down slowly, so that it would appear that they are flying. She never has her patients do more than ten repetitions of this exercise. Following this exercise, she has them rotate their arms so that their palms are facing upward, and they complete the same exercise. She calls this, "flying upside-down." Again, Leslee never asks her patients to do more than ten repetitions of this exercise.

The final exercise that Leslee asks of her patients is the tricep curl. In this she asks each patient to take the free weight in his or her hands and to first bring the weight above their shoulder on one side of their body in a set of ten repetitions. Then holding the weight out in front of them, she asks them to bring the weight in a downward arch behind them while keeping their arm bent. She asks ten repetitions of this exercise. Once they have completed this exercise with one arm, she asks them to complete it with their other arm. Once the patients have completed these exercises on both sides of the body, they have concluded the second part of Leslee's exercise program.

The final part of Leslee's exercise program is called, "cool down." She begins with what she calls, "the lazy man's exercise." It is a calming technique. While sitting in a chair, she asks her patients to bend their arms at the elbow and to bring their hands to the temporomandibular bone. She has her patients breathe in through their nose and out through their mouth slowly, while putting light pressure on their temporomandibular joint in a circular motion. She does this for one minute. Next she asks her patients to hug themselves to get proprioceptive input. After each patient is finished giving themselves a hug, she has her patients give themselves a pat on the back for completion of the program, to add a sense of accomplishment, and also to keep their shoulders loose. This ends Leslee's exercise program.

CHAPTER 3

Medical Terms Spoken in English

Alzheimer's Disease – The most common form of dementia. It is a progressive decline of brain failure with a seven to ten year course on average.

Vascular Dementia – Sudden onset after stroke. Risk factors are hypertension, smoking, vascular disease caused by diabetes. Within three months of a recognized stroke, deterioration and the progression of dementia is seen. The size and location of the bleed of the stroke determine what will be affected.

Multi-infarct dementia – Multiple strokes.

T.I.A.s- Transient ischemic attacks or little strokes.

Not Vascular Dementia – One lacunar infarct (i.e. small lesion–lunar or fingernail shape). Microvascular white matter changes of aging. Not a form of dementia. Strictly a stroke.

CVA – Cerebral Vascular Accident, or a stroke, can be caused by thrombosis, embolism or hemorrhage.

Hemorrhage – A bleed anywhere in the body. In the brain it can be very serious.

Thrombosis – A blood clot, again, anywhere in the body but usually located in the calf area. Very different from a spasm or cramping because it will appear red and sore and swelling is present.

Embolism – Some substance like air or fat travels into the blood vessel and blocks the airflow.

Deficit – Loss, or diminished ability, of the senses: movement, behaviors and personality.

Lesion – Interruption of function, which can be caused by the emboli blockage, a bleed or the blood clot.

Lewy Body Dementia – Slowly progressive dementia over six to ten years, with visual hallucinations and Parkinsonian symptoms such as tremors and rigidity.

Parkinson's Disease – A disease of the motor system. The brain is affected and causes ambulatory problems. Onset is typically after fifty with a gradual onset. Affects 2% of the population. 40% with Parkinson's Disease end up with Parkinson's dementia. 25% of Parkinson's patients have hallucinations. 33% of Parkinson's patients have depression.

Frontotemporal Dementia – Behavioral problems, a worsening of socialization, impulsiveness, very poor judgment. 40% of people with Frontotemporal Dementia have someone in their immediate family who also has Frontotemporal Dementia because of its high inheritance rate. The onset is usually around the age of 50 and the course of Frontotemporal Dementia generally takes ten years. Left-sided syndromes are prevalent, such as aphasia. Right-sided syndromes are also prevalent, such as behavioral disturbances.

Creutzfeldt-Jakob Disease – Mad Cow Disease or dementia. 90% die in one year. Caused by a protein that enters the brain and cannot be extracted.

Alcohol Induced Dementia – Wernicke-Korsakoff Syndrome.

Wernicke-Korsakoff Syndrome – Onset is early and causes much damage to the brain. Begins with short-term memory loss and ends with confabulation.

Confabulation – Lying to hide the fact that the patient does not know what they are talking about because of memory loss.

N.P.H. or Normal Pressure Hydrocephalus – Fluid on the brain, which has symptoms that can be reversed if caught in time. 50% can improve with early treatment.

AIDS – Related dementia, which can occur at any age with AIDS.

Aphasia – The inability to communicate, or a loss of the ability to verbalize or to understand what people are communicating to you.

Expressive Aphasia – The inability to communicate emotions and express one's self.

Receptive Aphasia – The inability to understand what another person is communicating.

Global Aphasia – Both expressive aphasia and receptive aphasia are present

Recognition – A memory disorder where lesion site would be in the thalamus of the brain.

Short-term memory – Found in the frontal lobe of the brain.

Long-term memory consolidated – In the thalamus and hippocampus or the limbic system.

Long-term storage – In the temporal lobe of the brain.

Long-term recall – In the temporal lobe of the brain.

Immediate Memory – A memory held consciously for less than one minute.

Short-term Memory – A memory held for more than a minute.

Long-term Memory – A memory held for more than a few minutes.

Recent Memory – A memory held for several hours or months and it overlaps with long-term memory.

Remote Memory – A memory held for many years; it can go back to childhood.

Episodic Memory – One's own personal history. An example of this was when one woman relived her son's death every day, as that was all that she could keep in her brain.

Verbal Memory – Memory of words and sentences.

Visual Spatial Memory – Memory of objects and spatial relationships.

Motor Memory – Memory of movement.

Sensory Memory – Memory of smell, taste, hearing, and visual experiences.

Emotional Memory – Memory which effects affect.

Apraxia – The inability to do learned movement functions in the absence of paralysis.

Constructional Apraxia – The inability to draw or accurately copy a model.

Dyskinesia – A behavioral state of disorganization.

Kinetic Apraxia – The inability to coordinate movement with parts of limbs, the inability to imitate another person's gestures.

Dementia – Permanent or progressive decline of intellectual function from normal social and economic activity.

A.D.L.s or Activities of Daily Living – Activities that a person does every day to care for himself and others.

Sensory Integration – Use of the environment as stimulation or to calm. With dementia patients calming sensory integration is used.

Blunted Affect – Refers to minimal facial expression or animation.

Constricted Affect – Refers to limited facial expression or

animation. Needing severe emotion to show any senti-
ment.

Flat Affect – Refers to the inability to show facial expression
or animations at all.

Labile Affect – Refers to rapid changes of emotion, such as
crying one moment and laughing the next, with wild, un-
predictable mood swings.

Delusion – False belief not shared by any family member or
anyone in their culture or religion.

Delusion of Grandiosity – The person has a special power or
talent, such as believing that they are Christ or Elvis Presley
or that they believe that they can read minds.

Delusion of Persecution – The person believes that they are
in danger.

Somatic Delusions – The person's believing that they have a
different diagnosis than they actually have. An example of
this is when a person with dementia believes that they have
brain cancer.

Hallucinations – A sensory thought with an absence of an
actual occurrence.

Auditory Hallucination – Hearing a voice or music that is not
actually there.

Visual Hallucination - Seeing a person, an animal, shapes, or
flashes of light that are not actually there.

Tactile Hallucinations – Belief that someone is touching
them when no one is actually touching them.

Olfactory Hallucinations – Particularly a belief that a
person has a particular body odor that no one else can
smell.

Illusion – Misinterpret shadows of people or noises.

Mood – Also known as affect. How is the patient presenting,
sad, overly happy, agitated, even aggressive.

Perseveration – Constant repetition of the same word, phrase or idea.

Pressured Speech – Rapid continuous speech that makes no sense and is often fragmented.

Word Salad – The person makes up words, is very incoherent and disconnected, making no sense at all.

Tardive Dyskinesia (TD) – Repetitive movement usually involving the mouth or the tongue, which is very rhythmical.

Adaption – According to Hirama (1987), an adjustment made so that a person can live more comfortably and more independently in their environment (31).

Integration – A meshing together of sensory work.

Praxis – The execution of body movement.

Proprioception – The position of the body in relation to another body part. An example of this is a person standing next to a chair, knowing and understanding that they are next to a chair.

Sequencing – Placing events and actions in order.

Vestibular – Balance.

Archaic Brain – The brain of snakes and lizards. Controls hunger, temperature, and fight or flight. The thalamus is found here. Our basic needs are met here, however, with dementia, if this area is affected, then hunger needs may not be met, for example, and the patient is never full and will continue to eat even when you try to stop them.

Old Brain – Or limbic brain. Cats and dogs have this type of brain and it is the subconscious brain. This system contains memory, mood and hormone production. Hippocampus is found in the old brain.

Hippocampus – Is the primary site of memory formation, or the nucleus or center of the old brain.

Amygdala – Controls our fight or flight response.

Hypothalamus – The major controlling organ of the endocrine system.

New Brain – Or the conscious brain. This is only found in humans. This controls our higher cognition. It allows us to have abstract thought, the use of tools, the ability to form and comprehend language and our social behavior. This is found in the frontal cortex or the frontal lobe. This is where dementia begins.

Neurotransmitter – Chemicals found in the brain that help it communicate with its various parts.

Acetylcholine – From the automatic nervous system regulation. It sends a signal from the nerves to the muscle and it aids in memory formation.

Neuroepinephrine or **Neuroadrenaline** – The lack of this chemical causes stress and depression. The presence of this chemical creates energy and increases hunger.

Dopamine – The presence of this chemical allows socializing, increases sex drive, and increases appetite and it also decreases hallucinations. The lack of dopamine causes hallucinations and lack of concentration. Dopamine is formed through exercise.

Seratonin – The presence of this chemical allows for the regulation of activity. It allows one to begin an activity, as well as to terminate an activity. Seratonin is formed through exercise.

Endorphins – The presence of this chemical allows a person to feel better about themselves and also acts as a natural form of morphine, in the way that it gets rid of the sensation of pain. Too many endorphins may not be healthy for a person. Endorphins are formed through exercise.

The Global Deterioration Scale – A scale that doctors can use in assessment of the level of a dementia patient, from level one of no cognitive decline, to level seven of very severe cognitive decline.

Brief Cognitive Rating Scale – A scale used to assess a patient by doctors, also used with the Global Deterioration Scale. This rating scale uses five axes to determine the level of cognitive decline. Axis I tests Concentration. Axis II tests Recent Memory. Axis III tests Past Memory. Axis IV tests Orientation. Axis V tests Functioning and Self-Care.

The Geriatric Behavioral Rating Scale – Another scale used by doctors to determine the level of deterioration in a patient with dementia. This scale includes wandering, verbal aggression, physical aggression, socially inappropriate or disruptive behavior, psychosis, resisting care, depression, and anxiety in its categories.

The Geriatric Depression Scale – Contains thirty yes/no questions. If a score of twenty or higher is obtained the patient is considered depressed.

Psychosis – A condition of the mind, which is characterized by an impairment of the intellect, and is the inability to perceive reality.

Wandering – A patient will wander constantly because of their fear and lack of understanding of their environment. This is caused by the "fight or flight" response and, if possible, the patient will escape their surroundings.

Mini-Mental State Exam – An exam with the maximum of thirty points testing the number of areas, from orientation through recall of the memory. The sections of the mini-mental state exam include orientation, registration, attention and calculation, recall, and language. There is controversy over what score would show impairment. Some believe that a score of twenty-one and below shows impairment, while others believe that a score of twenty-five and below shows impairment.

Visual Acuity – Determines how accurately a person can see objects.

Body Scheme – Internal awareness of how the body works.

Tactile – Touch.

D.S.M. – IV – The abbreviation of Diagnostic and Statistical Manual of Mental Disorders, fourth edition. It gives the symptoms of all psychological disorders.

Guardianship – Is the most effective benefit for a patient with medical issues, such as heart or stroke issues because the guardian can take care of all of the necessary medical issues with the exception of mental health issues. Done while patient is incompetent or does not have DPA.

Durable Power of Attorney – Is the most effective benefit for a patient with mental health issues because it allows for the person named under Power of Attorney to take over and make all decisions when the patient is mentally impaired, but the power of the person named under Power of Attorney can be revoked when the patient becomes well enough to make judgments again. Done while patient is competent and is able to have wishes known.

Power of Attorney – Handles financial and estate issues, but do not have much say in medical issues.

D.V.T. – Deep Vein Thrombosis, or blood clots mostly forming in the legs, as a result of poor circulation and a lack of water hydration. When a blood clot forms it hurts and the part of the body swells and becomes hot to the touch. If the blood clot breaks away and begins to move, the person will die within three minutes. If found before breaking away, blood clots are treatable with blood thinners.

CHAPTER 4

The D. S. M. – IV, Maslow and Erickson

Many family members are upset that their loved ones may need the facility that I work in. They may say, "Why is my mother in a locked unit?" The answer is that, even though this is out of character for her, she has dementia. The criterion for a demented patient to see a psychiatrist is based on the Diagnostic Criteria D.S.M. – IV. According to the D.S.M. – IV (1994):

"A) The development of multiple cognitive deficits manifested by both

    1) Memory impairment (impaired ability to learn new information or to recall previously learned information)

    2) One or more of the following cognitive disturbances:
        a) Aphasia (language distance)
        b) Apraxia (inability to carry out motor activity despite intact motor functions)
        c) Agnosia (failure to recognize or ID objects despite intact sensory functions)

d) Disturbance in executive function (planning, organizing, sequencing, abstract thinking)

B) The cognitive deficits in Criteria A1 and A2 each cause significant impairment in social or occupational functioning and represent a significant decline from a previous level of functioning.

C) The course is characterized by gradual onset and continuing cognitive decline.

D) The cognitive deficits in Criteria A1 and A2 are not due to any of the following:

1) Other central nervous system conditions that cause progressive deficits in memory and cognitive function (e.g., cerebrovascular disease, Parkinson's disease, Huntington's disease, subdural hematoma, normal-pressure hydrocephalus, brain tumor)

2) Systemic conditions that are known to cause dementia (e.g., hypothyroidism, vitamin B12 or folic acid deficiency, niacin deficiency, hypercalcemia, neurosyphilis, HIV infection)

3) Substance-induced conditions

E) The deficits do not occur exclusively during the course of a delirium.

F) The disturbance is not better accounted for by another Axis I disorder (e.g., Major Depressive Disorder, Schizophrenia) (85-86)."

An example of apraxia was when one patient refused to walk simply for no other reason than, "just because." She was very capable of walking. Moreover, she was only fifty-four years old. She made the choice to place herself in a wheelchair and to never walk again. Moreover, an example of agnosia would be for a patient to see a pen, but to identify it as a clock. An example of disturbance is when one patient insisted on wearing her under garment over her other clothing. The drugs used to help control the behaviors are familiar to psychiatry and I feel they should administer the drugs on this basis. I have seen some disasters when administered by PCP or well-meaning psychologists. This will probably get me in deep water with some of my colleagues.

Maslow and Erickson were two psychologists. Maslow believed in self-actualization in the hierarchy of needs, while Erickson believed in integrity versus despair. Erickson believed that putting life events and experiences in order would help a person come to an understanding and then find perspective in their life events. *Vital Involvement in Old Age* written by Erickson says that in our culture old age is a negative stereotype when it should be the best time of a person's life, or the grand finale, as it were. The cognitive and language impairments common with dementia cause old age to become more of a struggle than a grand finale.

In Maslow's Theory of the Heirarchy of Needs, fulfillment of needs and self-actualization are particularly important. According to Bowlby (1993) self-actualization (Maslow's term) is "an integrated understanding of who we are" (81). The fundamental need for a person with dementia is meeting those requirements so the self-actualization can happen, thus creating self-esteem. The next level is belonging and acceptance. By sharing life experiences, and having those encounters reaffirmed and accepted, a person arrives at personal accomplishment. This is where a caregiver's role is critical, because activity, (i.e., leisure activity, daily ADL schedules and life experiences), plays a crucial role in what a patient does. All of this creates the highest level of fulfillment, which is self-actualization.

CHAPTER 5

Memory

According to the D.S.M. – IV, written by the American Psychiatric Association (1994), dementia is an organic syndrome in which there is progressive deterioration of global cognitive functions, which impairs a person's occupational and social performance (85-89). The most common type of dementia is Alzheimer's disease. It is the fourth leading killer in the United States. When memory becomes impaired, all executive cognitive function is depleted.

There are three types of memory storage systems. These systems are the sensory (perceptual), short-term, and long-term memory systems. Memory is like a computer. The mind takes in information, stores it, and then retrieves it when needed. Similarly each part of memory has three stages. These stages include encoding, storage and retrieval. Encoding is imprinting information in the brain. Storage is maintaining the imprinted information so that it can be recalled at a later date. Finally, retrieval is accessing the imprinted information when it is needed.

The storage system has a very small capacity compared to the sensory perceptual system. It is limited to seven pieces of information, plus or minus two new pieces of information. This helps to narrow the information so that it is manageable, while also helping the brain to comprehend what is occurring outside of that information. To help the process of storage, people use their "chunking ability." "Chunking ability" groups pieces of information into smaller bits. An example of this is the social security number. According to Levy (web update) people are able to remember their social security numbers because they are grouped in three numbers, then two numbers, and then four numbers (web update).

Short-term memory lasts one second to thirty seconds. Most of short-term memory is lost when sights, sounds or thoughts distract a person. Activation memory is high when a person is paying attention, just as it is low when a person is distracted. The demented patient is easily distracted by their environment because of the fight or flight response, usually caused by a loud noise or the anxiety of being alone. To maintain information in short-term memory for longer than thirty seconds a person must use "maintenance rehearsal," which is the repetition of the information to oneself. Elaborate rehearsal is the capacity of working memory to organize information associated with other relevant information stored in long-term memory, so that it can be easily retrieved. An example of this might occur if a person is given a four-digit extension to a telephone number. Those four numbers are the same numbers as the last four digits in their sister's phone number. That person then makes the association between the extension number and their sister's telephone number, which allows them to store that information in their long-term memory. This technique can also be used for understanding meanings.

The hippocampus is the deep center of the brain and it is the primary site for long-term memory. Neuroscientists view the hippocampus as a switching station for short-term memory. If not for the hippocampus, most new connection and information would be lost.

The hippocampus has two forms of activation. The first form of activation occurs when the information perceived to have emotional significance is obtained. The second form of activation occurs when the information entering short-term memory is associated with stored long-term memory. These two forms of activation allow for the short-term memory to be saved as long-term memory.

Long-term memory is the largest component of information processing. It stores memories from a few minutes after they happened to very remote memories, which occurred a very long time ago. Activation is the process by which long-term memories are stored.

Encoding is a formation of abstract labels. [Primarily words with verbal labels and mental images, as well as auditory codes, and motor codes are formed into abstract labels.] According to an article written by J. Clark and A. Paviro (1991), our memory for images is better than our memory for words, which is why most of us remember faces more easily than names (3). One explanation is that pictures are stored in words and images, as well as being stored only as words.

There are two types of declarative memory, which include episodic and semantic, and one type of non-declarative memory, which is procedural. Episodic memory contains personal and relevant facts. Names, faces, birthdays, anniversaries, and where we left our keys are examples of episodic memory. Episodic memory is the least remembered part of memory. This is lost first in dementia patients because retrieval requires the ability to reconstruct events of the original experience.

Short-term memory consists of precise information, such as patterns of images, sounds and other sensory codes that the mind holds briefly and sorts consciously at any one time. This is conscious awareness or active memory. The information must be kept active in the short-term memory or it will be lost. Two sources of conscious awareness are processed in short-term memory. One source is sensory perception, in which a person would be able to consciously understand the identity of an object by a working knowledge in their long-term memory. An example of this would be a person understanding that a skunk does not smell pleasant, simply by looking at the skunk. The second source is information pulled from the long-term memory to help understand incoming information and ideas that are in a person's head at any given time. An example of this would be a person knowing that the gray object parked down the street is not an elephant, because they know from their long-term memory that it is a car.

Storage and processing is a very complex system. Two parts of this system are primary memory, which is storage for short-term memory, and working memory, which is trying to understand concepts while reading and retaining background information of what was previously read. Working memory is the process used for understanding language, engaging in planning and solving problems, and for decision-making and reasoning.

Encoding has three forms, which include images, semantic codes and sound. Most of the information in the short-term memory is encoded verbally.

Sensory perception memory is the first phase of intake of information from a person's surrounding environment. Environment stimulation (sights, sounds, smell, etc.) constantly affects our sensory perceptors. This information registers for four to five seconds, which is just long enough to be processed by our perceptual systems.

Encoding is sense specific in sensory perception. Nearly an exact replica of original sense is stored accordingly. The storing of visual sense is called iconic (icon) memory. Echoic (echo) memory is auditory sense memory and tactile (touch) sense memory. Sensory perceptional memory is huge because it stores all information provided by our senses, but because these memories do not last for a long time, they rarely interfere with the other parts of memory. Finally, paying attention to a perceptional memory and then sending it to short-term memory can retrieve information from sensory perception. If a person doesn't pay attention to the information it is forgotten.

Semantic memory builds on episodic memory, which involves knowledge and beliefs of facts and concepts without reference to where or when these originated (i.e., speaking language, planting and harvesting the garden). Semantic memory is complex, providing insight, knowledge and judgment. Semantic memory is retrieved with associated concepts and meanings in recognition of faces, body language and concepts of 3D spaces.

Procedural memory is the most long lasting memory. This type of memory even in later stages of dementia will remain. These memories are automatic, a motor response to environmental cues, such as reciting the alphabet, or peeling an orange or banana. They are efficient forms of cognitive function, while dealing with our surroundings automatically, with little thinking. At this point there is no standardized test for procedural memory. The procedural memory is implicit rather than explicit, as semantic and episodic memory are automatic, as well as dependent upon awareness. Implicit memory resides in the motor cortex and the cerebellum.

Episodic, semantic and procedural memory must be stored in an organized way. An important requirement of long-term memory is that the new information must be associated with information already stored in the long-term memory, so that it can be understood in the short-term memory. This involves elaboration, organization and environmental context addition of new meanings to existing knowledge in the long-term memory. Memories that are elaborated are changed to knowledge in that process and the knowledge is more easily retrieved later when it is needed at some future date. This process requires mental practices to keep the thoughts active. The more mental cues, the easier the retrieval. Moreover, information that is organized is easier to process and it is easier to store related information, especially if it is complex.

Environmental context works for episodic memory in particular. It is where a person remembers something by visual cues, or by retracing their steps. If a person is trying to remember the word spoon, it might be helpful for them to be in a kitchen. In patients with dementia, it is helpful for the person to see pictures of a setting to help them. For example, a patient seeing a picture of a bathroom may find it easier to participate in toileting.

Stored memory must be retrievable to be useful. Only a small area of the cerebral cortex is activated at one time; therefore, over-stimulation of the memory can cause anxiousness in dementia patients because recall memory is affected. Recognition involves association; therefore, recall memory is more taxing. However, if the right cues are provided (i.e., physical, psychological and environmental) the appropriate behavioral response can be reached.

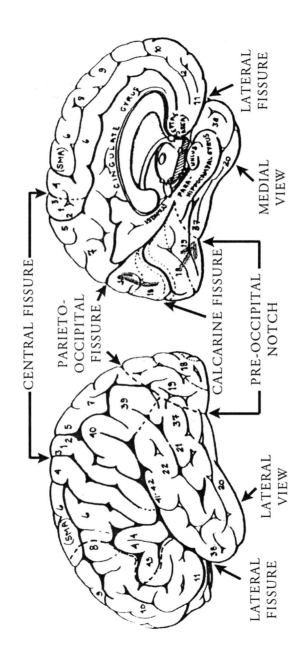

FRONTAL LOBES

Prefrontal Lobes: (9, 10, 11, 12) Judgement (foresight and hindsight) with relation to emotional tone, motivation and memory.

Premotor Cortices: Anticipates, plans and programs skills (including speech, body language, visual movements and survival strategies): Premotor Cortex (6), Supplementary Motor-Speech Area (6), Frontal Eye Fields (8), and Broca's Motor-Speech Area (45-44).

Motor Cortex: (4) Executes skills (including speech and body language) and survival strategies.

PARIETAL LOBES

Sensory Cortex: (3, 1, 2) Receives "raw data" from somatosensory input via the thalamus and relays multisensory signals to adjacent areas.

Sup. Parietal Lobule: (5, 7) Appreciation of senses, compares with past experiences in relation to stereognosis, body image, visual-spatial perceptions and movement detection. Functions with Inferior Parietal Lobule.

Inferior Parietal Lobule or Supra-marginal and Angular Gyri: (40, 39) Symbolic language and communication, especially reading, writing and arithmetic.

OCCIPITAL LOBES

Visual Cortex: Adjacent to Calcarine Fissure (upper and lower 17). Receives "raw data" from visual input via the Lat. Geniculate Nucleus of the Thalamus.

Assoc. Visual Cortices: (Adjacent areas or upper and lower 18 and 19.) Functions with Parietal Lobes and Post. Temporal Lobes in understanding what is being seen (Central Vision) and context (Peripheral Surround) and compares with past knowledge.

TEMPORAL LOBES

Auditory Cortex: (41-42 in Lat. Fissure). "Raw data" of auditory input via the Thalamus.

Assoc. Auditory Cortex or Wernicke's Area (22-21): Understanding of auditory input, compares with past knowledge and experiences.

Inferior Temporal Lobe: (37, 20) Visual-object recognition (persons, places and things); colors; relationships of objects; compares with past experiences. Ant. Temporal Lobe: (38, 20 in part).

LIMBIC CORTEX

Limbic Cortex: Septal Area, Cingulate Gyrus, Isthmus, Parahippocampal Gyrus and Hippocampus, Uncus and Amygdaloid Nucleus: Functions with all other cortices especially Prefrontal-Ant. Temporal Lobes and Hypothalamus: memory circuits, motivation, olfaction, visceral and emotional tone, fear and frustration, anger, rage, violence continuum and behaviors.

CHAPTER 6

Phase One—
The Pre-diagnosis

Phase One of dementia, or the pre-diagnosis, is categorized by many signs and symptoms. During the period of pre-diagnosis, a patient will begin to find that they are becoming forgetful or having early confusion. There is often a forgetfulness of names, events, or phone numbers. Also, a person may become disoriented or lost in familiar surroundings. For example a person might be driving home from work, a task that they have done for the last 30 years, and they make a right turn instead of a left turn. In some cases, they might not be able to remember exactly where home is.

A person experiencing Phase One of dementia may also exhibit signs of depression. This occurs in the later years of life and without a prior history of depression. Conetreras, Vargas, Ramos, and Velandia (2006/2007) reported that, "depressive symptoms occur frequently in patients affected by [dementia]. . . . Research suggests that individuals presenting a first depressive episode in adult life might develop dementia three to eight years later. Some authors suggest that depressive reactions could be early signs of dementia" (411). It is important to note, however, that much of what looks like depression is actually the inability to make executive decisions, which makes a person seem much more inert than they might otherwise be. Moreover, a person with Phase One of dementia realizes that something is wrong with them when they become disoriented or forgetful, or when they find that they are having trouble making decisions and that instills a fear in them. That fear, compounded with the difficulty in making decisions and the lack of spontaneity that also accompanies Phase One of dementia, all help to add to what appears to be depression.

Another characteristic of Phase One dementia is that the person may become easily angered or irritable. This may also be caused by their inability to make decisions and their realization that something is wrong. The person is usually completely aware of their losses and may express concern over their lost abilities.

Phase One dementia also creates a problem for a person in spatial awareness; this in turn creates a problem in knowing where the body is in space (proprioception). There is a test called the Clock Drawing Test in which a patient is asked to draw a clock. There is usually a problem with their spatial perception and so their drawing of the clock is a poor representation of an actual clock. Then the patient is asked to draw the hands of the clock at a specific time, for example 3:45. The patient will be unable to draw the hands at the time 3:45. Paskavitz, Gunstad, and Samuel (2006/2007) stated, "Clock-drawing tests are sensitive to executive dysfunction and are recommended as a screen test for cognitive impairment in [dementia]" (454). This test is a great indicator of pre-diagnosis dementia.

There was a male patient brought into the Geriatric Mental Health Floor for depression at the age of 65. During a group activity, which was a creative expression group, the male patient chose to draw a clock. His clock was an example of the type of clock a person with pre-diagnosis dementia would draw. The clock was spatially distorted with the numbers jammed up and there were numbers placed out of order. His clock even included the number twelve twice and also, the number thirteen. He placed no hands on his clock at all. This was the indication that this man was not suffering from depression, as had been previously thought, but that he was instead suffering from Phase One of dementia.

The patients in Phase One dementia may find that they have olfactory hallucinations. These hallucinations are the instances of smelling smells that are not actually real. An example of this would be a person thinking that they smell body odor when there is no apparent body odor. This is caused by changes to the brain, which are a product of dementia. According to Conetreras, Vargas, Ramos, Velandia (2006/2007), "In pre-clinical [dementia], there are already structural changes in the limbic system and neocortical brain regions, and some depressive symptoms may reflect early changes in brain regions critical to the ability to allocate and sustain attentional energy" (411). The limbic cortex has a prefrontal lobe, anterior temporal lobes and the hypothalamus. It functions with all other cortices of the brain. The limbic cortex controls the memory circuits, motivation, the sense of smell, and emotion tone. When the limbic cortex is structurally changed, feelings of fear and frustration may become very strong and there may be olfactory hallucinations. Moreover, when the limbic cortex is structurally changed the memory circuits will not work as they normally would, and that is when disorientation and forgetfulness can occur. The limbic cortex works with the prefrontal lobes, the premotor cortices, the motor cortex, the sensory cortex, superior parietal lobule, inferior parietal lobule or supra marginal angular gyri, the temporal lobes and the occipital lobes. The prefrontal lobes control judgment, emotion tone, motivation, and memory. The premotor cortices anticipate, plan, and program skills for speech, body language, visual, and survival. The motor cortex controls executive functions such as speech and body language, as well as survival. The sensory cortex controls somatosensory input via the thalamus. It relays multisensory signals. The superior parietal lobule compares past experiences in relation to body image, visual spatial, and movement detection. The inferior parietal lobule, or supra marginal angular gyri, controls symbolic language, communication and reading, writing and arithmetic. The temporal lobes can be broken down into the auditory cortex, associate auditory cortex and Wernicke's area and the inferior temporal lobe. The auditory cortex controls auditory input via the thalamus. The associate auditory cortex and Wernicke's area control understanding auditory input and compares it with past knowledge and experience. The inferior temporal lobe controls visual recognition of person, places, or things, color, and relationships of objects. The occipital lobes contain the visual cortex and associate visual cortices. The visual cortex and associate visual cortices function with the parietal lobes and posterior temporal lobes to understand what is being seen and to compare it with past experiences. This includes central and context vision. In order for a person to be fully functional all parts of the brain must be working together and structurally sound. In the event of the limbic cortex, or any other area of the brain, being structurally changed, the other cortices of the brain may fail to function properly.

CHAPTER 7

Phase Two—Early Dementia

P hase Two of dementia, also known as Late Confusional–Early Dementia, is characterized by many traits and behaviors. During phase two of dementia, a patient will begin to revert back to an earlier language. Their vocabulary will begin to diminish to words with only one to two syllables. Though a Phase Two dementia patient knows what they are attempting to express, their language skills are lacking and so their language becomes much less sophisticated. They will also be unable to do word-finding problems and have difficulty following a storyline. In the event that a story would be told to a patient in Phase Two, they would not be able to repeat the storyline, but they would attempt to manipulate the people around them, so that they would think that the patient was able to repeat the storyline.

Along with other losses, in Phase Two of dementia abstract thinking, such as planning and problem-solving are impaired. A patient with dementia will notice their inability to solve problems, and this will cause a great frustration in them. They are fully conscious of their lost abilities.

Patients in Phase Two of dementia also forget routine tasks, such as personal grooming and the rules of driving. Initially, in the first phase of dementia a patient forgot things like how to get to their house from work, which is something that they might have known for twenty-five years or more, but in the second phase of dementia a patient forgets much more. They may forget to bathe themselves for over a week, despite the fact that their normal schedule was to bathe themselves every other day. Or a patient with Phase Two dementia may forget to change their underwear. Their lack of personal hygiene causes increased body odor, which becomes noticeable to those around them. Although a patient with dementia may forget to practice personal hygiene, they do not realize it. In their reality, they believe that they have been showering and changing their underwear on a regular basis and so the difference of what is reality and what they believe to be reality often breeds paranoia and suspicion. Also, because patients with Phase Two of dementia are neglecting themselves, they may make complaints of neglect, because they honestly believe that healthcare staff, or their families or friends are neglecting them. Moreover, Phase Two patients often forget other routine tasks, such as the rules of driving. This is particularly scary considering the number of demented people driving around the country. When a demented person forgets the rules of driving they may run red lights, drive through stop signs, or forget to obey the speed limit, which increases the possibility that they may cause a traffic accident.

A patient with Phase Two of dementia may also lose or misplace items, but rather than admitting that the items are lost, they believe that the items have been stolen. This is in part because of the paranoia that exists as a product of reality versus their reality. Patients with Phase Two of dementia honestly believe that someone is out to get them in one form or another, and the person that their paranoia is usually directed toward is a family member or close friend.

As with people with ADHD, or attention deficit hyperactivity disorder, patients with Phase Two of dementia also have shortened attention spans. They are very easily distracted. This is a common characteristic of Phase Two of dementia.

Patients with Phase Two of dementia often resist help with activities of daily living. For example a patient who has not bathed for a long period of time will not allow someone else to help them bathe. Often the patient does not bathe because they have a fear of water flowing over their face and they have forgotten how to breathe when water flows over their face. A caregiver may provide the option of a basin bath, which will clean the patient just as well as a shower might with the exception of cleaning the hair the way that a shower would. Moreover, a basin bath would prevent water from running down the patient's face, however, the patient cannot understand that a basin bath would clean them without having water run down their face and so they refuse the help of the caregiver. This is often a result of their problem-solving impairment.

Patients with Phase Two of dementia have decreased ability to handle finances as well. Although, they may have balanced their checkbook or kept track of their credit card limits and amount spent for decades, when early dementia sets in the patient is incapable of doing these things. It is normal for patients with early dementia to do wild things with their finances, like not paying bills, thinking that they paid bills that were never paid, or hiding money as a result of their paranoia and then forgetting where their money is hidden. Usually, family members are blamed for stealing money that was misplaced or lost by the patient, or family members are blamed for unexplained overages in a checking account, which occurred because the patient forgot to pay a bill.

Moreover, the anxiety that a patient in Phase One of dementia displays is increased in Phase Two of dementia. The anxiety grows as the losses grow. The patient understands that they are losing their ability to function as they had functioned before and it causes heightened anxiety to the point of panic attacks.

In the second stage of dementia patients often begin to wander. This is a result of being restless and impatient. Patients who wander usually forget where they are and are lost. Often they are wandering as an attempt to escape because they feel trapped. This is most common at sundown because the light changes and they want to get home to their husbands or to their wives or to their families.

Denial is a common coping skill among Phase Two patients of dementia and their families. They are not ready to admit that they have dementia and that they are forgetting things. Moreover, patients of Phase Two usually do not want anyone to know that anything is wrong with them, so they will attempt to hide their dementia by manipulating the people around them. In a few cases, the patient's denial is so strong and their social skills are intact and they are capable of convincing people around them that there is nothing wrong with them. In most cases, a patient's social skills remain through Phase Two of dementia.

I have heard many a family member say, "This will get better with the medication right?" At the moment it is only a temporary fix and, no, this is just the tip of the iceberg, but you and your demented relative do not need to sink with the Titanic.

CHAPTER 8

Phase Three—Middle Dementia

During Phase Three of dementia, or Middle Dementia, even more changes take place in a patient. The patient's gait changes. Where they used to walk normally and be able to keep up a brisk pace, now they move in small and halting steps. In addition to their gait change, their wandering increases. This is caused by the fight or flight response. When the patient gets to the point where they are trying to escape (or take flight) from their familiar surroundings, they begin to wander. If allowed out of the house, they become a danger to themselves because there is more of a chance that they may fall and be hurt, or that they will wander into an unfamiliar place and be lost. In one case, a woman wandered out of her home and into the woods. Her body was found two months later.

Also, patients in Phase Three of dementia experience increased rigidity. The increased rigidity is a result of a combination of incorrect functioning of the brain, apraxia, and fear. With fear the muscles of the body tighten. Moreover, the brain is not functioning properly at this point. It becomes unable to process the command for smooth movements. Finally, there is apraxia. Apraxia is decreased ability for purposeful movement. The patient's motor skills begin to deteriorate and their movement control begins to fail. Tasks as simple as picking up a spoon or fork are now nearly impossible for these patients. It becomes much easier for them to eat with their fingers than with utensils.

With Middle Dementia, a patient will also have bowel and bladder incontinence. It is often at this point that a caregiver becomes unable or unwilling to continue care of the patient and so the patient is sent to a nursing home or an assisted living facility. More than likely a patient at this stage will end up in a nursing home, unless they still are able to complete some of their activities of daily living, such as walking, feeding themselves, and dressing themselves. If the patients are still able to perform their activities of daily living, they are suitable to be placed in a locked assisted living facility. However, most assisted living facilities are very expensive and most insurance pays a minimal amount or not at all.

Patients of Middle Dementia will also experience a decreased ability to read and do math. Along with this they will experience aphasia. Aphasia is the decreased ability to understand and express language. Aphasia is the step past echolalia. Echolalia is a singsong pattern of certain words, sounds or phrases that usually rhyme, used in repetition. Aphasia is the point where a patient wants to say something, but they no longer have the words to get across what they are trying to say. Usually they will find a phrase that gets them attention from the people around them and that is the phrase or word that they will use in repetition. Moreover, with aphasia, patients have trouble comprehending larger words, and so they might need to have sentences broken down into smaller words. It is important for a caregiver to constantly ask questions such as:

"Do you need to use the bathroom?" "Are you hungry?" "Do you want water?" "Do you want juice?" These questions are simple enough for a patient to understand and they can usually communicate an answer well enough to the caregiver to receive what they need.

Along with apraxia and aphasia, patients with Phase Three of dementia also experience agnosia. Agnosia is the decreased ability to recognize objects. A patient with agnosia would not be able to recognize an apple, a penny or a table if they were shown these objects. When shown an apple, a patient with agnosia might say that it is a pencil. However, when the agnosia is very bad the patient will not be able to identify the apple and so they will not say anything at all. In the event that a tea cup set on a saucer with a spoon were set in front of the patient, they would simply stare at it, unable to know what to do with it. They would not know what the saucer or the spoon is. Moreover, coupled with the apraxia, the patient would be unable to pick up the teacup from the saucer. In this event, the caregiver should place the teacup into the patient's hands, where it will become familiar to them and they will drink from it.

During Middle Dementia a patient might experience perseveration. Perseveration is a thought or thought pattern that repeats itself for a certain amount of time. This thought pattern is then vocalized when the patient uses one or more of the words in the thought in a repetitious cycle. The patient's thought might be, "Help me." However, they can only manage to say the word, "Help," and so they repeat it until the thought is no longer stuck in repetition in their brain. This is a cycle that could last for fifteen to twenty minutes before it is broken (the broken record). Moreover, patients with Middle Dementia often actively resist help with ADLs or activities of daily living. As with Phase Two patients, certain ADLs such as showering or brushing one's teeth may scare the patient; how-ever, the fear of ADLs increases and so the patients of Phase Three more actively resist help in those activities. It is rare that a patient with Phase Three of dementia would be persuaded and helped to bathe by a caretaker more than once in a week.

Along with resisting help with ADLs, patients of Phase Three of dementia also display aggressive behaviors. This is part of their fight or flight response. They will hit, kick, scratch and bite people who they do not remember. The first in their memory to be lost are usually grandchildren. After they forget their grandchildren they begin to forget their own children. The last person that a person with Middle Dementia forgets is their spouse, although they may continue to trust this person, or confuse them with a parent. In the case of a family member who has been forgotten visiting the patient, they may display an aggressive behavior toward that family member because they are angry.

Moreover, the affect of a patient with Middle Dementia is flat or blunted, or lacking emotion. When someone looks into the eyes of a person with dementia, they will notice that the eyes are completely emotionless. In the case of a blunted affect, the entire face of a patient with Middle Dementia will be emotionless and look as though there is no tone in it.

With Phase Three of dementia, the paranoia and agita-tion of the patients increase. A patient may become very frus-trated and agitated because they are trying to express them-selves, but are unable. Moreover, when a patient forgets their family members their paranoia increases. They may be in a room with their son, whom they no longer recognize and sud-denly in their head they are in a room with a stranger. Another example of paranoia occurred when a patient said that a man was stealing all of her money. The man that she thought was stealing her money was her husband and he was using their money to pay the bills.

Finally, patients with Phase Three of dementia begin to have hallucinations, delusions and confabulation. The most common are visual hallucinations. Visual hallucinations of little people stealing things from the patient are very common; however there are a broad variety of possible hallucinations. A patient might experience auditory hallucinations, or tactile hallucinations as well as visual hallucinations. With tactile hallucinations a patient might believe that someone has just touched them when they have not been touched at all. Moreover, with auditory hallucinations a patient might believe that they just heard someone say something to them when there was no sound around them. Also, the patient may experience confabulation, which is when they begin to tell lies as part of their survival instinct. It is manipulative language. When asked how many children the patient has, they may not remember. When asked to name their children, they may give actual names of their children, but then they will give names that are not the names of their children in an attempt to appear as if they do know all of the names of their children. This is confabulation. Moreover, a patient of Phase Three of dementia will experience delusions. A patient may have delusions of grandeur in which they believe that they are wealthier than they actually are. However, as with hallucinations there are many different types of delusions that a patient might experience.

CHAPTER 9

Phase 4—Late Dementia

During the final stages of dementia, Phase Four or Late Dementia, a patient is in the final stage of their life. Phase Four does not last very long. Generally, the patient's loss of the rest of their bodily functions characterizes Late Dementia. Before immobility, patients often have slowed movements. Patients then become non-ambulatory, which means that they can no longer walk. When a patient becomes immobile, the problems associated with immobility persist. These problems include the breaking down of the skin, and bedsores. Patients, on average, must be turned and propped every two hours to keep their skin from breaking down once they become immobile.

A loss of the ability to communicate verbally is also a characteristic of Late Dementia. Words are completely lost to a patient and they may begin to scream, or they may fall entirely silent. With the loss of the ability to communicate, a patient becomes completely isolated from everyone else, so it is important for the caregiver to attempt to integrate them into social activities and programs to ease the isolation.

Seizures also accompany Phase Four of dementia. The brain deteriorating and the breakdown of the neurotransmitters cause these seizures. Also, a lack of oxygen could cause seizures.

In Late Dementia swallowing problems, or dysphasia, also persist. Dysphasia occurs when the patient forgets to swallow. Most patients are given thicker liquids to help prevent aspiration. Aspiration occurs when liquid or food enters the lungs. In a person without dementia, liquid or food entering the lungs may not be such a serious problem because they are active and able to cough out whatever entered the lungs. However, for a patient with late dementia who is no longer mobile, food and liquid entering the lungs becomes a terrible problem because they are unable to rid themselves of the food or liquid and it can create an infection in the lungs. Aspiration of liquids is the most common form of aspiration in patients of Late Dementia. It is comparable to drowning because they slowly take water into their lungs as a result of their dysphasia.

Also, during Phase Four of dementia, a patient also begins to experience loss of body weight. This occurs because the body itself is preparing for death. Loss of body weight is one of the final things that happens before a person passes away. When a patient with Late Dementia passes away it is common that their brain forgets to tell their heart to beat, or that they aspirate and die. Also, patients with dementia may stop breathing because their brain forgets to tell them to breathe.

Hospice is recommended for this stage of dementia, as it is a fast-moving stage of dementia, and the last stage before death. Patients in this final stage usually no longer eat and drink of their own choice, and so they can sometimes be kept hydrated intravenously. However, it is painful to a patient to be hydrated in this manner and so at this point, as they are prepared to pass away, hospice care is a recommended option.

$\mathcal{A}ctivities$

T here are different levels of activity groups for patients with dementia. The different groups are parallel groups, project groups, egocentric-cooperative groups, cooperative groups and mature groups. These different groups function at varying levels. While a parallel group functions at a level appropriate for a patient whose dementia has gotten to the Middle Stages, a mature group functions at a level that would not be appropriate for patients who are not extremely high functioning.

A parallel group is the group that would be more appropriate for low-functioning patients with dementia. Within a parallel group patients are made comfortable, so that they will not feel threatened, thus eliminating the fight or flight response. A parallel group engages the patient into interactions with others on a very limited basis, offering them a task that is a task the entire group is conducting, but treating that task as though it is an individual task, specific to each person of the group.

A project group is a group that is still appropriate for low-functioning patients with dementia; however, it can also be used as a group for higher-functioning patients with dementia. In a project group patients engage in group activities, though they are allowed to enter and leave the group activity as they wish. With low-functioning patients, a caregiver may give them pieces of blue construction paper and ask them to rip it into smaller pieces to be used for a bulletin board project. While with higher-functioning patients, a caregiver might ask patients to cut up green construction paper with scissors, or to glue the blue and green pieces of construction paper together. In this way patients are asked to perform tasks at their appropriate levels, while being integrated socially with each other.

In an egocentric-cooperative group patients are usually higher-functioning patients with dementia. Egocentric-cooperatives are social groups. According to Mosey (1973), patients in these groups are "aware of [the] group's goal relative to the task" (92). Moreover, they enjoy participating in the group. Most of the time the patient is eager and willing to participate and will act as a part of the group. Also, socially, a patient who takes part in an egocentric-cooperative group recognizes and respects social norms and the rights of others. Also, according to Mosey (1973) usually these patients "[meet] the esteem needs of others and [are] able to [have] others [in the group] meet his [or her] esteem needs" (92). The egocentric-cooperative groups are highly social groups for the higher functioning patients.

A cooperative group is a group for extremely high-functioning patients with dementia. In these groups patients who are not of an extremely high level of functioning would most likely experience a fight or flight response. In these groups patients are able to respond to each other in a very respectful and social manner. This is because the patients are functioning at a level in which they are conscious of their own wants and needs and they are concerned with the wants and needs of the people around them. However, a patient in this group is most likely to gravitate toward a patient who is similar to them in one way or another.

In a mature group, patients with dementia would not be able to take part. Mature groups are meant for people who have no cognitive deterioration. There are occasions where patients in the earliest stages of dementia may participate in a mature group. In these groups a person must be able to respond to all group members. Also reported by Mosey (1973), people in a mature group must be able to undertake "a variety of task roles" (92). It is imperative that a group member be able to understand and carry out the task, which they are assigned. Moreover, a person in this group must be able to satisfy the task given, while also satisfying the needs of the group members around them. Mosey (1973) also wrote that it is important for a person in a mature group to have more than one perspective and to take "a variety of social-emotional roles" (92). In interacting with other group members a person must be sensitive and sympathetic to those around them. In the event that a person would be unable to handle different social-emotional roles, they would not be able to fully participate in a mature group, thus mature groups are generally not used for patients with dementia.

Creative expression groups are groups utilizing artwork. This type of a group is appropriate for all levels of dementia. It can be modified to do simple paper tearing, to painting, to cutting with scissors. A caregiver can give one-step tasks and even assist with the task. Or a caregiver can give multiple-step tasks, without assistance. The creative expression groups are meant to be used to help patients express themselves. A patient could take out their frustrations by tearing paper, or they could feel a great sense of accomplishment in themselves for completing a task. Creative expression groups also allow for social interaction by allowing a patient to sit within the group of people, or by allowing a patient to carry on a conversation with other patients who are capable of conversations.

A baking group is a purposeful group. This group helps a patient continue doing something that they have been doing all along, such as making food. This type of a group can incorporate patients with all levels of dementia, by handing out appropriate tasks to patients. Moreover, there is a social aspect to this group as well. Also, this group encourages reminiscing by allowing a patient to remember food that they've enjoyed their entire lives. A patient might smell muffins baking and be struck by a memory of cooking with their mother or their grandmother as a child. Patients are encouraged to share their memories with the group to promote socialization in a non-threatening environment.

Sensory work is a group utilizing as many senses as possible without over-stimulating the patient. This group is usually used for Middle Stage to End Stage dementia patients, and is helfpul to calm the patients. These groups are kept very small and are an example of parallel groups. The lighting is kept low. A patient may be sat in a rocking chair and allowed to look at a picture book with no words. This is soothing to them and sitting in the rocking chair aids with the patient's balance. Moreover, a picture book does not challenge the patient, but allows them to look at something aesthetically pleasing, which may help to trigger occasional memories.

Animal assisted therapy, or an animal assisted group, can be used with all levels of dementia. In this group emotion is evoked in the patient simply by sitting with the animal, even at a non-verbal stage of dementia. In higher-functioning patients with dementia, there is a more social aspect to this type of therapy. Often they reminisce and share their memories with each other. These patients are encouraged to pet the animal, which must be trained as a therapy animal. The petting of the animal gives the patient a sensory experience as well.

A sing-along group can be a challenging group, because over-stimulation of patients can occur. If the music is too loud or the group becomes too rambunctious a patient may become overly stimulated, which is why this group must be very closely controlled. A sing-along group can be great therapy though. In a sing-along group, patients may not be able to remember the words of the songs, but the songs can still evoke emotions from them, and bring back memories from earlier times in their lives. In this way, patients in a sing-along group can relieve their stress and release their emotions.

Relaxation groups are for high-functioning patients. In early stages of dementia, a relaxation group gives the patients coping skills. If the coping skills are repeated enough a patient may be able to use them to the point of moderate dementia.

Leslee also has a relaxation activity that she conducts for her patients. She suggests that the relaxation activity should be conducted at the calmest time of the day for the patient or the caregiver. This activity, when completed correctly, should take ten minutes. She has her patients sit in a chair with their shoulders loose. Each person does the deep breathing exercises, by breathing in through the nose and out through the mouth. As they breathe in their belly should go out and as they breathe out their belly should go in. During this breathing exercise she asks her patients to close their eyes and concentrate on a number if they are capable of focusing on a number. If the patient is able to focus on a number she suggests that they begin with the number two hundred and work backward to the number one. If the patients are not capable of focusing on numbers, she asks her patients to focus on a ball of color, that is either dark purple, dark green or royal blue. If the patients are not capable of focusing on a ball of color either, she plays soft music by Debussy in the background. A patient may fall asleep. In the instance that a patient falls asleep, they should not be allowed to sleep for more than thirty minutes because it will interfere with nighttime sleep.

Leslee also conducts a progressive relaxation technique for her highest-functioning patients. She asks her patients to clench their toes for ten seconds and then to unclench their toes for ten seconds. She has her patients do ten repetitions of this exercise. Next she asks her patients to tighten their ankles for ten seconds and then to loosen the ankles for ten seconds in repetitions of ten. She moves up the body to the knees, the thighs, the buttocks, the fists, the arms, the shoulders, the teeth and the eyes in succession. She asks the patients to tense each body part for ten seconds and then to loosen for ten seconds in ten repetitions. If done correctly, this exercise should take ten minutes. It helps the patients to concentrate on the task instead of concentrating on their stressors, which puts them at ease and relaxes them. If a patient becomes too frustrated with this relaxation technique, the first relaxation activity, deep breathing, should be used.

Another exercise that Leslee conducts is called, "The Lazy Man's Exercise." She conducts this exercise for patients that she sees becoming frustrated. After isolating the patient she has the patient sit in a chair and she asks them to close their eyes and to concentrate on their breathing. The patient is asked to bend their arms at the elbows and to place the hands on their temporomandibular joint and to rub that joint in slow circles while continuing to breathe deeply. This loosens the muscles in the face and the neck, increases blood flow and redirects the patient's frustrations. At the end of this exercise the patient should be calm and relaxed. According to Leslee, "The Lazy Man's Exercise" redirects the patient's focus and they begin to use this exercise as a coping skill. This exercise is the fastest relaxation, coping skill that Leslee practices.

If a patient becomes over-stimulated and is unable to be calmed by any of these techniques, they should be isolated to a quiet corner with no stimulus around them. There should be no noise, no music, no movement, no activity, nothing to distract their attention in this corner. If the patient is acting out, but is capable of listening to the caregiver's voice, the caregiver may try to calm the patient with a soothing tone. However, if a patient is acting out and is incapable of listening to the caregiver's voice, it is encouraged that the patient be left alone in complete quiet of the corner with no stimulus.

Finally, Leslee recommends that patients participate in gardening groups. In these groups she suggests that the patient be able to deal with the many stimulations that come from the sensory integration of gardening. She suggests that plants and flowers with aromas be used because the scents and aromas of the plants and the flowers create a conversation piece for the patient and the caregiver. Moreover, the smell of a flower or an herb may bring the patient back in time to a memory of their youth. Also, gardening can be adapted to suit each patient. If able, patients may garden outside; however, gardens may also come inside in the form of tabletop potted plants. Some patients prefer herb gardens, while others enjoy bright flower gardens. Each patient is different and the variety that gardening offers has the potential to meet each patient's needs and offers them a social and calming activity.

CHAPTER 11

Environment

The environment in which a patient with dementia is living is very important. An environment could either hurt or help a person with dementia.

In a living room, the room should be free of clutter, allowing room for a walker. It should have chairs that are easy to get in and out of, with high backs and arms. Also, a living room should not have throw rugs and all cords should be behind furniture, so that the patient does not trip and fall. A living room should always have the correct lighting, which can be turned on at the entrance of the room. Also, in the living room, there should be a cordless phone so that if a person were to slip and fall they could use the phone to call for help.

In the kitchen, the room should be very basic. There should be trays of food for patients so that they can continue to self-feed. In patients with lower-functioning dementia, there may need to be trays of finger food. Self feeding is very important. Give one item of food at a time and one utensil and the person can eat independently. Also, there should be correct lighting. As in living rooms, there should be no throw rugs or cords that can be tripped over. In a kitchen, microwave ovens can be used by patients with dementia; however, there should always be oven mitts and potholders right by the microwave oven, so that the patient does not burn themselves on overly hot plates or foods.

The bathroom is the most dangerous room in the home. The bathroom is a place where a patient with dementia is most likely to fall and be hurt. To minimize the chances of a fall, always keep a rubber mat inside of the tub, as well as outside of the tub, unless there is wall-to-wall covering. Also, install grab bars so that the patient can hold onto the bars when getting on or off of the toilet. A raised toilet seat is also important. Finally, a cordless phone should always be kept in the bathroom so that if a patient were to slip and fall and hurt themselves, they could use the phone to contact help.

In the bedroom always have the clothing easily accessible for the person. Always keep one season of clothing available to the person. If there is a caregiver, the caregiver should place the outfit for the patient to wear in a designated place to minimize the amount of confusion over choices. Also, there should be no throw rugs in the bedroom and no cords that can be tripped over. A cordless phone should also be kept in the bedroom. A great place to keep a cordless phone is directly beside the bed. Also, if the patient needs a cane or a walker, the cane or walker should be kept directly within reach to the person from the bed. Moreover, a lighted path should be made from the bedroom to the bathroom.

Medication bottles should be labeled with large enough letters that the patient can read the bottles without glasses. Also, if the patient is in Stage One or Two of dementia, they can still use a pillbox. The best type of pillbox for a patient in Stage One or Stage Two of dementia is the seven-day pillbox that is split into morning and afternoon of every day, thereby making each pillbox have fourteen compartments. It is important, however, to make sure that a person with dementia does not overdose on their medications because this could cause delirium, which could worsen the dementia of that patient.

CHAPTER 12

Sensory Integration

Sensory integration is a tendency to react or not to react to the stimulus in the environment. Most people will not be adversely affected or react to these environmental stimulus. Over-sensitivity to light, unstable surfaces, high frequency noises, visual stimuli and smells can result in stress, anxiety, or behavioral patterns that develop in an attempt to cope with what they perceive as irritations within their clothing and environment. Sensory stimuli have the power to do two things: either alert a person or calm a person. With proprioception in geriatric patients, light to deep pressure on their body are better suited than light touch because light touch could over-alert them, while light pressure calms them. Also, in regards to the vestibular system with geriatric patients it is important to move the patient slowly, not quickly. If the patient needs to be taken in the opposite direction, they should not be spun around to face the opposite way quickly, but they should instead be taken around in a large circle, slowly. According to a report by Kinnealy, Oliver, and Wilbarger (1994) in regards to the tactile system with geriatric patients it is important to remember to use soft textures, instead of using harsh or abrasive ones, because harsh and abrasive textures could irritate the patient (444-451).

Sensory integration comes from work developed by A. Jean Ayres, PhD., OTR. Her research was done with children. However, if you look at the dysfunction in children with difficulty in sensory integration and dementia patients, the similarities are extraordinary. Hatch-Rasmussen (1995) wrote that when observing children using tactile, vestibular and proprioceptive stimuli, which they consider to be the building blocks of sensory integration. It was observed that tactile dysfunction is shown by refusing to eat certain foods, isolation in social settings, distractibility and hyperactivity. Hatch-Rasmussen (1995) also stated that dysfunction in the vestibular system manifests itself in difficulty walking on uneven surfaces, climbing stairs, and fearfulness in space. Dysfunction in proprioception is exhibited by a tendency to fall and eating in a sloppy manner. Dysfunction with motor planning is another form of dysfunction in proprioception. This manifests as language and speech delays, impulsiveness in a new environment, and withdrawal appearing as depression. Using sensory integration functioning and the ability to repeat ADLs will re-occur.

In a study with the elderly, patients were asked to take a quiz screening knowledge and available social support. The next year more tests followed and orally administered tests were given the following year. The study showed a decrease in depression due to chronic pain because of the use of sensory integration. According to Phillips' (2000) report the only difference in treatment with matched control groups was the use of sensory integration.

A report from Baker, Dowling, Wereing, Dawson and Asseg (1997) stated that Snolzelen, meaning "Snuff and Dose," consists of plausible sensory experience. It is effective in reducing cognitive demands and after ten minutes the calm remains (213-218).

Studies have shown the same behavioral problems shared between autistic and demented patients. Kinnealy, Oliver and Wilbarger (1994) reported that three studies dealing with sensory integration in adults show that lack of sensory input interferes with choices of activity, ADL and increase in the time taken to avoid fearful situation (444-451). An example of this might occur if there were too much noise surrounding them, and people with dementia opted to isolate themselves socially, or refused to leave their house. In the instance of the glare of sunlight, a person with dementia could not be convinced to wear a hat and sunglasses to go out; instead they would refuse to go outside altogether. Also, a person with dementia experiences changes in their taste buds and for this purpose they refuse to eat foods that they used to enjoy. They may refuse to eat certain foods because of the way that the foods feel in the mouth in a tactile sense. Finally, with dementia patients the olfactory system is the first system to be affected by dementia, and so the patient may believe that they have body odor even when they don't and for that reason, they may isolate themselves from other people.

CHAPTER 13

Case Studies

THE CLOCK GUY:

T his man came to the mental health unit for depression. He was still able to do his ADLs, make his food, drive his car, etc. During one of the sessions a therapist had him draw a clock. It was by his clock drawing that the mental health unit was able to identify that he was in the earliest stages of dementia. He was immediately placed into the program for patients with dementia.

In order to help this patient the staff of the mental health unit had him complete puzzles, word searches, art projects and other activities that challenged his brain. Also, they had him exercise. He also learned to do new non-threatening activities, which kept his brain functioning at a higher level. These activities greatly helped the clock guy.

THE MIDDLE AGED WOMAN:

There was a woman who began to exhibit signs of dementia in her late fifties. She would repeat herself. An example of this is when she would give a recipe to someone and then fifteen minutes later she would repeat the same recipe to the same person. Her dementia took ten years to run its course. Eventually, this woman gave up traveling with her husband because she became too afraid. In the end, she gave up her entire life and every social aspect of her life. Had she continued to socialize she would have prolonged her life.

JEAN:

Jean is in the early moderate stage of dementia. She is still able to complete her ADLs without help. However, she is beginning to have communication breakdowns. She has begun to wander about the mental health unit. She becomes very anxious when there is too much verbal stimulation. Also, when she is around other anxious patients she becomes more anxious and frustrated.

Jean helps to complete chores like clearing tables. She also enjoys completing jigsaw puzzles. Also, she participates in exercise groups and word groups at her level. Because socialization is difficult in groups with Jean, the mental health staff uses a parallel group to help Jean. Moreover, she is given a pillowcase so that she may wander about and gather objects. She puts the objects inside of her pillowcase and at the end of the day when she goes to bed the staff returns all of the objects to their rightful homes so that Jean can wander and gather the same objects the next day. Jean also enjoys reminiscing, though she is very protective of her personal space.

THE MARINA LADY:

The Marina Lady had moderate dementia. When the mental health staff met this woman she still had her expressive verbal skills, though she had receptive aphasia. Also, she was unable to perform her ADLs. She needed help with bathing and dressing. The staff would initiate and terminate a task and this woman would complete the portion of the task between initiation and termination. In eating, the staff would break down this patient's tray of food to one food, one utensil and one napkin. Once The Marina Lady finished the food in front of her, the staff placed the next food in front of her. This was to minimize her confusion over the food before her. If too many foods were placed in front of her she would stare at the foods, unable to eat any of them. Also, The Marina Lady enjoyed reminiscing. She was delusional in her environment. The Marina Lady always thought that she was in a marina enjoying a few drinks with the staff members talking to her. She was a former alcoholic. Moreover, the more that she reminisced, the more anxious this woman became. Eventually, the staff came to realize that while this woman was sitting in the marina on a beautiful day enjoying a few drinks with her friends, she had let her six-year-old son drown. Every day this woman relived the day that her son had died, but it wasn't until the staff saw her relive the full memory that they realized that she was reminiscing about something terrible. It was at this point that the staff learned that not all reminiscing is positive. It was important for the staff to learn to redirect The Marina Lady, and to restructure her reminiscing to a place where she would be less anxious. The staff began to redirect The Marina Lady's reminiscing from the marina, to New York City because they had learned that she used to take many trips to New York City. In this way they still encouraged her reminiscing, but they kept her reminiscing positive.

The Marina Lady also sat down in a wheelchair one day, though it happened to be for no apparent reason. The staff realized that if The Marina Lady continued to stay in the wheelchair, that her dementia would be hastened by the lack of exercise. The nursing staff at the hospital conducted themselves by using reality orientation, in which they would use reality as a stimulant; however, the mental health staff recognized that reality orientation is not always the answer. In the case of The Marina Lady, she was searching for her dead husband. Instead of telling this woman that her husband had passed away, the staff of the mental health unit encouraged her to get out of the wheelchair by using her husband. They told this woman that if she left her wheelchair she might be able to find her husband more quickly than if she stayed in her wheelchair. After working with her for nearly an hour the staff had convinced The Marina Lady to leave her wheelchair. She was about to stand up and take a step when a nurse entered the room from the hallway and said to The Marina Lady, "But dear, your husband is dead." This caused The Marina Lady to give up hope of finding her husband, which gave her no purpose to leave the wheelchair. In the end, not only did The Marina Lady stay in her wheelchair, but she also began to grieve the loss of her husband again. She was unable to be sent to an assisted living facility and was instead sent to a nursing home, where because of lack of exercise and hastened dementia, she passed away six months later.

It was by The Marina Lady that the staff of the mental health unit learned that they couldn't redirect this patient to reality, but that they must instead go to the reality of the patient. If a patient is stuck in their past, the staff should meet them in the past instead of trying to redirect them to the present.

THE THREE MUSKETEERS:

These patients were in their early sixties and they were near the end stages of their mental processes. All of these patients had the same physical appearance, though they were not related. In appearance they were reminiscent of the cartoon of Droopy Dog, in the sadness in their faces. They were no longer able to initiate, terminate or complete their ADLs. Also, they appeared to be in a constant stage of fight or flight. Whenever the staff would attempt to do a group activity they would become agitated and run away in their fight or flight response. In order to keep them calm the staff needed to reduce all of the stimuli in their environments. Also, the only way that these patients became comfortable in a social setting was to stand with their foreheads against the wall without moving. Though a member of the staff of the mental health unit felt like a failure in the case of these three patients, she realized that they needed to stand with their foreheads against the wall without moving because that was what was best for them.

LEROY, THE KING:

Leroy liked to be in control of things, even in his late dementia. He no longer ambulated. He was using a wheelchair. Moreover, Leroy spent more time sleeping than awake. However, when he was awake Leroy was able to exercise his body to a certain degree. In his past, Leroy was a very intelligent man, so when his family members or staff members of the mental health unit came to him with a task he would become very frustrated and he would scream like a banshee. Before Leroy became demented he was very controlling of his family members, and so his family members became passive-aggressive. In his dementia, his family members attempted to control Leroy and so he would lash out in his agitation and he would scream and yell in an attempt to control his family members. Also, Leroy ate breakfast and dinner, but he refused to eat a lunch, which greatly upset his family members. The staff of the mental health unit fed Leroy a liquid lunch to keep him hydrated so that he wouldn't get delirious and they then counseled Leroy's family. In fact, Leroy's family received more counseling than Leroy because Leroy was unable to comprehend much verbal speech. As Leroy's family stopped pushing Leroy to do things that he didn't want to do, he began to exhibit a sense of humor with a twinkle in his eye.

THE SCREAMING LADY, THE WORST CASE SCENARIO:

This is a case where family denial and not dealing with dementia at the beginning stages of dementia can allow terrible things to happen at the end of the dementia. This woman was diagnosed at a very early stage. She was able to walk about, socialize, perform her ADLs and she went to groups. She enjoyed art. Also, she participated in exercise groups, though she did not always want to participate. She enjoyed the animal-assisted therapy as well.

This woman's dementia progressed to the point where she was unable to perform her ADLs by herself. The staff of the mental health unit had to terminate and initiate her ADLs for her and they helped her feed herself. Her speech had more expressive and receptive aphasia. Moreover, she went from being able to walk with a walker to having to sit in a wheelchair because she fell and broke her hip. All through this portion of her life, her family was in denial, which hurt this woman's situation.

From the break of her hip, this woman needed surgery. She was given general anesthesia, which hastened her dementia. Moreover, despite the fact that this woman was able to walk again, the pain in her hip never left her, so she opted to spend her time in a wheelchair because of her inability to understand the need to walk would reduce her pain.

This woman forgets to feed herself, and she begins to forget to swallow. She also aspirates into her lungs, which causes pneumonia. Her family attempts to force her to eat, but because she has forgotten to swallow she pockets her food in her cheeks. Moreover, she begins to scream because she is in pain from her hip and from her lungs. Even at this point, her family believes that she will make a full recovery.

Finally, after doctors, nursing staff, activities staff, and social workers tell the family that this woman will not make a full recovery, they agree to put her in hospice, however, the family insist that she is given IV fluids. Because of the IV fluids The Screaming Lady did not die in one week, as she should have, but instead lived for three weeks. The staff of the mental health unit had to allow this woman to go on in the state that she was in because there was no durable power of attorney due to the family's initial denial over The Screaming Lady's condition. Eventually the family acquired a durable power of attorney. They could have prevented weeks of suffering for their mother and themselves if they had faced the facts, as difficult as that was. It takes a lot of strength.

.

CHAPTER 14

Books and Articles Worth Reading

Bowlby, C. (1993). *Therapeutic Activities with Persons Disabled by Alzheimer's Disease And Related Disorders.* Gaithersburg, MD: Aspen Publishers.

This book was written specifically for adults in regards to sensory integration. Chapters four and seven are the favorite chapters of Leslee Wlodyka.

Advance for Occupational Therapy Practitioners. November 29, 2004, Vol. 20, No. 24, "Reducing Caregiver Burden."

This article gives a great detailed narration of how to adapt a house so that it will be a safe environment for patients with dementia.

Richeson, Nancy, PhD., CTRS. (2003). Effect of Animal Assisted Therapy on Agitated Behaviors and Social Interactions of Older Adults with Dementia. *American Journal of Alzheimer's Disease and Other Dementias*, 18(6).

This article is exceptional because it shows the true statistics of positive social interaction and the decrease of agitation in demented patients with the use of animals in animal-assisted therapy.

––––––––––––

Heyn, Patricia, PhD. (2003). The Effects of a Multisensory Exercise Program on Engagement, Behavior, and Selected Psychological Indexes in Persons with Dementia. *American Journal of Alzheimer's Disease and Other Dementias*, 18(4).

This article discusses the benefit of exercise on patients with dementia. While the exercise regimen discussed in the article is a little more advanced than the exercise program done by Leslee Wlodyka, it is still an excellent program, and the article about the program is informative.

––––––––––––

Horst, Goran, PhD., RNT., Ingalill R. Hallberg, PhD., RNT. (2003). Exploring the Meaning of Every Day Life for Those Suffering From Dementia. *American Journal of Alzheimer's Disease and Other Dementias*,18(6).

This article should be read because it shows the shame, sorrow and sadness of patients with dementia and it shows each person's need to be treated as an individual.

––––––––––––

Small, Jeff A. PhD., JoAnn Perry PhD., RN, Julie Lewis, MSC. (2005). Perceptions of Family Caregivers Psychosocial Behavior When Communicating With Spouses Who Have Alzheimer's Disease. *American Journal of Alzheimer's Disease and Other Dementias*, 20(5).

This article is very important reading material because it helps a person understand the relationship between psychosocial attributes of a caregiver's behavior and communication outcomes for persons with Alzheimer's and spousal caregivers. In this article a person learns the correct way to address a person with Alzheimer's.

Hodder, Ruth. (2004). Vignettes Connections: My Gateway to a World of Silence. *American Journal of Alzheimer's Disease and Other Dementias*. 19(2).

This is a good article because it is from a daughter's point of view and it shows how Alzheimer's can bring families closer together if allowed. It directs the reader to look at the positive aspects of Alzheimer's, rather than dwelling on the negative aspects.

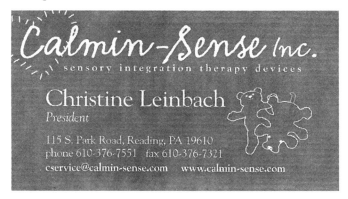

Bibliography

American Psychiatric Association. (1994). D.S.M. – IV.

Arkin, S. *American Journal of Alzheimer's Disease and Other Dementias.* Vol. 22, #1, Feb./Mar. 2007, pg. 62.

Baker, R., Dowling, Z., Wereing, L.A., Dawson, J., & Asseg, J. (1997). Snolzelen: Its Long-term and Short-term Effects on Older People with Dementia. *British Journal of Occupational Therapy*, 60(5), 213-218.

Bowlby, C. (1993). *Therapeutic Activities with Persons Disabled by Alzheimer's Disease and Related Disorders.* Gaithersburg, MD: Aspen Publishers.

Clark, J., & Paivio, A. (1991). *Educational Psychology Review.* Vol. 13, #3.

Conetreras, Vargas, Ramos, Velandia. *American Journal of Alzheimer's Disease and Other Dementias.* Vol. 21, #6, Dec. 2006/Jan. 2007, pg. 411.

Hatch-Rasmussen, C. (1995). *Sensory Integration.* Retrieved from the Web 10/18/2001. http://www.autism.org/si.html

Heyn, P. (2003). The Effects of a Multisensory Exercise Program on Engagement, Behavior, and Selected Psychological Indexes in Persons with Dementia. *American Journal of Alzheimer's Disease and Other Dementias*, 18(4), 248.

Hirama. H. OT Assistant Activities A Primer 1996 update.

Kinnealy, M., Oliver, B., & Wilbarger, P. (1995). A Phenomenological Study of Sensory Defensiveness in Adults. *American Journal of Occupational Therapy*, 49(5), 444-451.

Levy, MD, Norman B. http://ajp.psychiatryonline.org/cgi/content/full/159/10/1804.

McCarthy, B. (2000). *About Learning.*

Mosey, Anne Cronin OTR, PhD, FAOTA Activities Therapy, 1973 Raven Press Books Ltd.

Paskavitz, Gunstad, Samuel. *American Journal of Alzheimer's Disease and Other Dementias.* Vol. 21, #6, Dec. 2006/ Jan. 2007, pg. 454.

Phillips, R.S.C. (2000). Preventing depression: A Program for African American Elders with Chronic Pain. Retrieved from the Web 10/10/2001. http://www.findarticles.com/cf_0/m0F-SP/4_22?58576053/print.html

Teri, L., McCurry, S.M., Bucher, D.M., Logsdon, R.G., La-Croix, A.Z., Kukall, W.A., Barlow, W.E., & Larson E.B. (1998). Exercise and Activity Level in Alzheimer's Disease: A Potential Treatment Focus. *Journal of Rehabilitation Research and Development*, 35(4), 411-419.

Voltz, Raymond. (2005). *American Journal of Alzheimer's Disease and Other Dementias.* Vol. 19. http://www.medscape.com/medline/abstract/10869059?prt=true.

Printed in the United States
145713LV00001B/83/P